THE CLEAN GUT HANDBOOK FOR MEN AND WOMEN

THE A-B-C TO RESTORING YOUR GUT HEALTH AND VITALITY

By

Dr. Chris Allan

Copyright @ 2023 Chris Allan
All rights reserved

Table of Contents

Dr. Chris Allan

INTRODUCTION

Picture a life where you wake up energized, free from bloating and discomfort, and ready to take on the day with vitality. Imagine bidding farewell to those afternoon slumps and finding relief from stubborn weight gain that just won't budge. The secret to transforming your well-being lies within your gut – that intricate ecosystem of micro-organisms that holds the key to overall health.

In these modern times, our bodies are constantly bombarded by pollutants, stressors, and processed foods laden with hidden additives. It's no wonder that more and more people find themselves battling fatigue, digestive issues, and a weakened immune system. The key to reclaiming your vitality and achieving a state of true wellness lies in understanding the remarkable power of your gut.

Drawing on the latest research in gastroenterology, nutritional science, and holistic wellness, this handbook is meticulously crafted to provide you with a comprehensive roadmap to a clean and rejuvenated gut. Prepare to embark on a journey that will not only cleanse and heal your intestinal system but will also revitalize your entire body.

Inside the "Clean Gut Handbook," you will discover:

The Gut-Body Connection: Uncover the intricate link between your gut health and overall well-being. Learn how a compromised gut can affect your immune system, mental clarity, skin health, and more.

Nurturing Nutrition: Explore a curated list of gut-loving foods that will supercharge your healing process. Say goodbye to bloating and discomfort as you embrace a wholesome and delicious approach to eating.

Holistic Habits: Dive into a treasure trove of holistic practices that go beyond diet. From stress-reduction techniques and sleep optimization to mindful movement, these habits will support your gut on every level.

Gut-Healing Recipes: Revitalize your kitchen with a collection of recipes designed to banish inflammation and cultivate a thriving gut environment. Discover easy-to-follow dishes that prioritize taste without compromising your health.

Your Personalized Plan: Every individual is unique. Learn how to tailor your approach to gut health based on your specific needs and preferences. This handbook will empower you to design a sustainable wellness journey.

The "Clean Gut Handbook" is more than just a guide—it's a transformative tool crafted to empower you with the knowledge and resources needed to embark on a life-changing path towards optimal health. Get ready to awaken your body's inner healing power and unlock a new-found vibrancy that radiates from within. Your journey to a clean gut and a revitalized life begins now.

CHAPTER ONE

THE GUT-HEALTH CONNECTION

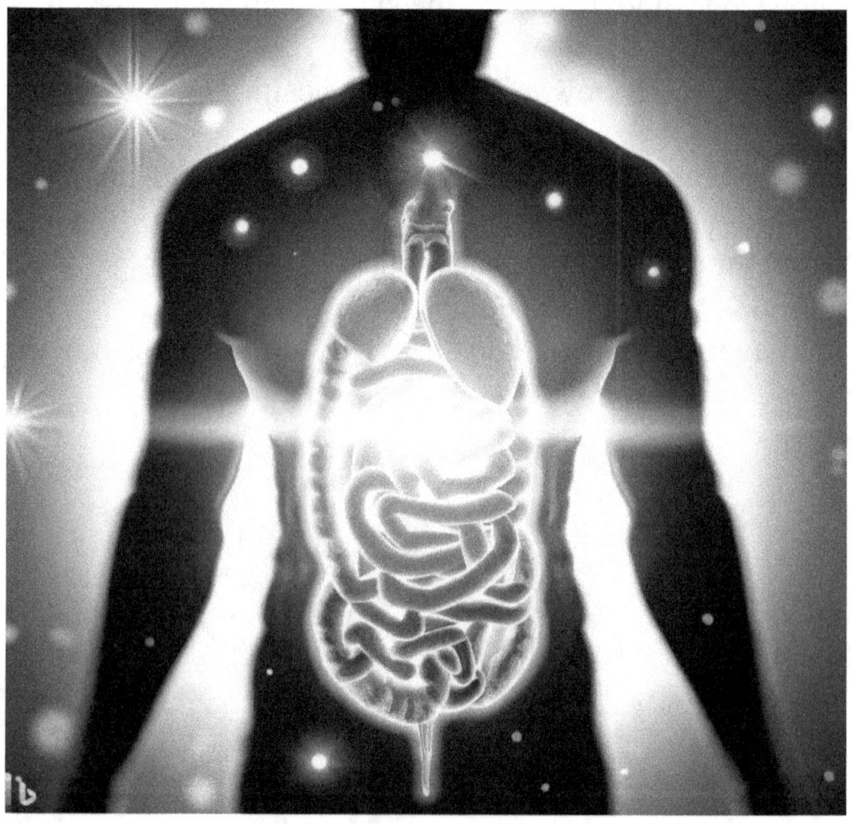

In the vast expanse of the human body, a thriving world exists, teeming with an unimaginable diversity of life. This world, invisible to the naked eye, is the gut microbiome, a complex and enchanting ecosystem that plays a symphony of roles, influencing not only our physical health but our mental well-being as well. As we embark on a journey of exploration into this microcosm, we unveil the profound interconnectedness that shapes our very existence.

Picture, if you will, a bustling cityscape under a microscope. A kaleidoscope of micro-organisms, ranging from bacteria to viruses, fungi to archaea, form a labyrinthine metropolis within our intestines. This living tapestry, collectively known as the gut microbiome, is as intricate as the galaxies above, with each microbe contributing its unique melody to the grand orchestration of life.

The gut, often hailed as the "second brain," is not merely a vessel for digestion. It is a crossroads where science and art intertwine, and where the molecules of sustenance meet the dance of evolution. This ecosystem, which has evolved over millennia, is a testament to the profound adaptability of life itself. Yet, only in recent years has science lifted the veil on its secrets, allowing us to explore its enigmatic depths.

Within this inner cosmos, countless species coexist in harmony, forming a delicate balance that sustains us. Just as a rainforest thrives with diversity, the gut microbiome thrives on it. The bacteria in our intestines outnumber our own cells, and their genetic material dwarfs our own. This realization humbles us, reminding us that we are but a small part of a much larger narrative.

The intrigue of the gut microbiome lies not only in its numbers but in its impact. It is a maestro that conducts the symphony of our health, influencing digestion, metabolism, and even immune response. It crafts a harmonious melody that resonates through our bodies, sculpting the contours of our physical well-being.

Beyond the tangible, the gut microbiome extends its influence into the ethereal realm of emotions and thoughts. Recent studies have unveiled an astonishing link between gut health and mental health. The gut-brain axis, a highway of communication between the two, opens avenues for emotional landscapes to be painted by the microbes residing within us. The delicate balance of the microbiome can shape our moods, influence anxiety and depression, and even steer the course of neurological disorders.

As we voyage further into this uncharted territory, we marvel at the therapeutic potential that lies therein. The gut microbiome, once an unexplored frontier, now holds promise in fields as diverse as personalized medicine, nutrition, and psychology. It has the power to transform our understanding of health and disease, offering novel solutions to age-old challenges.

Yet, as we delve into this microcosm, we must tread with humility and respect. The delicate equilibrium of the gut microbiome is easily disrupted by our modern lifestyles, marked by antibiotic use, processed foods, and stress. In our quest to unravel its mysteries, we must remember that our actions shape this ecosystem and, consequently, our own well-being.

In the grand theater of existence, the gut microbiome is a masterpiece in the making. As we uncover its complexities, we uncover a deeper truth – that we are intricately woven into the fabric of life, intimately connected to the cosmos within and around us. The journey into the gut microbiome is not merely a scientific exploration, but a pilgrimage to the heart of what it means to be alive. So let us venture forth with wonder and reverence, for within us lies a universe waiting to be discovered.

LINKING GUT HEALTH TO OVERALL WELL-BEING

In the intricate tapestry of human existence, a silent conductor orchestrates a symphony of health and vitality that often goes unnoticed - the gut. Nestled within us, the gut harbors a vibrant ecosystem of micro-organisms that wield an astonishing influence on our physical, mental, and emotional well-being. Beyond its role as a mere digestion center, the gut is an intricate nexus, interconnecting seemingly disparate aspects of our lives into a harmonious whole.

Picture the gut as a lush garden, teeming with a diversity of flowers, each representing a strain of microbes that play an integral role in shaping our health. Just as a skilled gardener cultivates a balanced environment to ensure vibrant blooms, nurturing a diverse and balanced gut microbiome is essential for our well-being. When this microbial symphony is in tune, the effects ripple outward, touching every facet of our lives.

Physically, the gut microbiota is a guardian of our immune system, acting as an army that shields us from invaders and keeps inflammation at bay. But its influence doesn't stop there. Emerging research unveils a profound connection between gut health and mental health. The gut-brain axis, a bi-directional communication pathway, demonstrates how the gut and brain engage in constant dialogue. Imagine neurotransmitters as messengers traversing this axis, carrying news of mood, stress, and emotions. When the gut microbiome is balanced, this communication flourishes, contributing to emotional equilibrium and resilience.

Consider moments of "gut feelings" or "butterflies in the stomach" before an important decision. This is more than mere metaphor – it's a reflection of the intimate connection between the gut and intuition. The gut's enteric nervous system, often referred to as the "second brain," is an intricate web of neurons that operates independently, yet in tandem with the central nervous system. This second brain not only governs digestion but also influences our emotional state, response to stress, and even social interactions.

As we delve deeper into the fascinating world of the gut, we unveil a profound revelation: the gut microbiome has the power to shape our cravings, impacting our dietary choices and thus, our long-term health. A well-nourished garden will yield bountiful produce; similarly, a nourished and diverse gut microbiome encourages healthy food choices, promoting overall well-being.

However, in the modern age, our microbial garden is under siege. Factors like processed diets, antibiotics, and chronic stress can disrupt the delicate balance, leading to a symphony in disarray. The consequences are far-reaching - from digestive distress and weakened immunity to mood disorders and chronic diseases. Yet, hope lies in our hands. By embracing a holistic approach to health, we can cultivate our inner garden, sowing the seeds of well-being.

Nurturing gut health is a multifaceted endeavor. A diet rich in fiber, fermented foods, and a rainbow of plant-based nutrients serves as fertile soil for beneficial microbes. Mindfulness practices, meditation, and stress management compose the nurturing sunlight that helps our gut flora flourish. Additionally, an active lifestyle cultivates an environment where diverse microbes thrive, enhancing nutrient absorption and toxin elimination.

In essence, the gut is not merely a humble bystander in the grand play of well-being. It is the quiet maestro, conducting a profound concerto that resonates through our bodies, minds, and spirits. To recognize the pivotal role of the gut is to embark on a journey of self-discovery, where the foods we eat, the thoughts we think, and the environments we inhabit are all threads woven into the fabric of our vitality.

So, let us embrace the wisdom of our gut, for in doing so, we embrace the essence of holistic well-being. As we care for our microbial garden, we nurture a profound connection to ourselves, our surroundings, and the symphony of life that dances within and around us.

CHAPTER TWO

ACCESSING YOUR GUT HEALTH

Each organ in the human body plays a special part in preserving balance and harmony, creating a complex symphony that is the body. The gut is a conductor among them, managing the complicated dance of digestion, absorption, and immunological protection. This symphony may be disrupted by an unhealthy gut, resulting in a discordant song that vibrates throughout the body. The signs and symptoms of an unhealthy gut are like whispers, subtle yet revealing, guiding us to delve deeper into the realm of our well-being.

Digestive Distress: The Symphony Out of Tune

Digestion is a meticulous process that involves multiple organs and an array of enzymes working in perfect synchrony. An unhealthy gut can throw this harmony off balance, resulting in digestive distress. Symptoms may include bloating, gas, constipation, diarrhoea, and even heartburn. These whispers often signify underlying imbalances in gut bacteria, inflammation, or compromised intestinal lining.

Food Intolerances: The Unheard Cries

When the gut's delicate lining is compromised, it can lead to the leakage of substances into the bloodstream, triggering immune responses. This can manifest as food intolerances or sensitivities. The body's reaction to certain foods, such as gluten or dairy, can be a telling sign of an unhealthy gut. Paying attention to these whispers can help identify potential triggers and provide insights into gut health.

Mood Swings and Mental Well-being: The Gut-Brain Connection

The gut and brain share an intricate relationship often referred to as the gut-brain axis. A distressed gut can send signals to the brain, affecting mood and mental well-being. Anxiety, depression, irritability, and even brain fog can be linked to an unhealthy gut. Understanding and nurturing this connection can be pivotal in achieving holistic wellness.

Skin Signals: A Mirror to Gut Health

The skin, the body's largest organ, can mirror the health of the gut. Conditions such as acne, eczema, or psoriasis might be whispers from the gut, indicating inflammation or imbalances. A deeper exploration of gut health could unveil solutions that go beyond topical treatments, addressing the root causes of these skin concerns.

Weight Fluctuations: The Gut's Role in Metabolism

Maintaining a healthy weight involves a complex interplay of factors, including metabolism. An unhealthy gut can influence the body's ability to regulate weight, potentially leading to unexplained weight fluctuations or difficulties in shedding excess pounds. Listening to these whispers can guide individuals toward strategies that encompass not only dietary changes but also gut-focused interventions.

Chronic Fatigue: When the Gut Drains Energy

Fatigue that persists despite adequate rest is another whisper that might indicate an unhealthy gut. The gut's role in nutrient absorption and energy production is significant. An imbalanced gut can compromise these functions, leaving individuals feeling perpetually drained.

Acknowledging this whisper could unveil the path to renewed vitality.

Autoimmune Clues: Unravelling the Immune System

Research suggests a strong link between gut health and autoimmune conditions. An unhealthy gut can trigger an over-active immune response, potentially leading to autoimmune diseases. Signs such as joint pain, inflammation, or unexplained allergies might be the gut's way of signaling underlying immune imbalances.

The signs and symptoms of an unhealthy gut are not mere nuisances; they are the body's whispers, guiding us toward a deeper understanding of our well-being. Embracing these signals and embarking on a journey to restore gut health can yield profound benefits that extend far beyond digestion. As we unravel the mysteries hidden within these whispers, we gain the power to reclaim our health and rewrite the symphony of our lives in harmonious melody.

DIAGNOSTIC TOOLS AND TEST

A harmonious balance of micro-organisms residing in our gastrointestinal tract contributes to proper digestion, nutrient absorption, immune system regulation, and even mental health. As the scientific community delves deeper into the intricate interplay between gut health and various aspects of human physiology, an array of diagnostic tools and tests have emerged to shed light on this hidden microbial universe.

1. Microbiome Analysis: Unlocking the Microbial Diversity

The centrepiece of modern gut health diagnostics is microbiome analysis. This revolutionary approach involves studying the composition and diversity of the gut microbiota, which includes bacteria, viruses, fungi, and other micro-organisms. High-throughput sequencing technologies, such as 16S rRNA gene sequencing and meta-genomic sequencing, enable researchers and healthcare professionals to identify and quantify these microbial inhabitants.

2. Stool Tests: A Window into Gut Health

Stool tests, also known as faecal tests, have long been a cornerstone of gut health diagnostics. These tests provide valuable insights into the presence of pathogens, levels of beneficial and harmful bacteria, and markers of inflammation. They are particularly useful for diagnosing conditions like irritable bowel syndrome (IBS), inflammatory bowel disease (IBD), and infections.

3. Digestive Function Tests: Unravelling Enzymatic Activity

Digestive function tests assess the efficiency of various enzymes and processes crucial for proper digestion and nutrient absorption. One common example is the pancreatic elastase test, which measures elastase levels in the stool to evaluate pancreatic function. These tests aid in identifying conditions such as pancreatic insufficiency.

4. Food Sensitivity Testing: Navigating Dietary Triggers

Food sensitivity tests help individuals pinpoint specific foods that may trigger gastrointestinal discomfort, inflammation, or other symptoms. While controversial in some circles due to variable accuracy, these tests analyze blood or stool samples for antibodies or other markers associated with adverse reactions to certain foods.

5. Hydrogen and Methane Breath Tests: Unmasking Carbohydrate Mal-absorption

Hydrogen and methane breath tests are non-invasive procedures used to detect malabsorption of certain carbohydrates. During digestion, gut bacteria ferment undigested carbohydrates, producing gases like hydrogen and methane. Elevated levels of these gases in breath samples can indicate conditions such as lactose intolerance or small intestinal bacterial overgrowth (SIBO).

6. Gastrointestinal Endoscopy: Direct Visualization

Gastrointestinal endoscopy allows healthcare professionals to directly visualize the gut lining using a flexible tube with a camera attached (endoscope). This technique aids in diagnosing conditions like ulcers, polyps, and gastrointestinal bleeding. Advanced versions, such as colonoscopy and upper endoscopy (esophagogastroduodenoscopy), offer comprehensive assessments of the colon, small intestine, and stomach.

7. Calprotectin and Lactoferrin Tests: Assessing Inflammation

Calprotectin and lactoferrin are proteins released by white blood cells during inflammation. Tests measuring these proteins in stool samples can help distinguish between inflammatory conditions like Crohn's disease and ulcerative colitis versus non-inflammatory disorders.

8. Gut Permeability Tests: Gauging Intestinal Barrier Function

Gut permeability tests evaluate the integrity of the intestinal barrier, which prevents unwanted substances from entering the bloodstream. An impaired barrier has been linked to conditions ranging from autoimmune diseases to allergies. These tests often involve measuring the presence of specific molecules (e.g., zonulin) in blood or urine.

In the rapidly evolving field of gut health diagnostics, these tools represent a mere fraction of available options. As researchers deepen their understanding of the gut's role in health and disease, innovative methods for assessing gut health continue to emerge. From microbiome analysis unveiling the intricate web of micro-organisms to advanced endoscopic techniques providing a visual panorama of the gastrointestinal tract, these diagnostic tools empower healthcare professionals and individuals alike to embark on a journey of gut health optimization. Ultimately, these tools not only aid in diagnosis but also serve as a compass guiding us toward personalized strategies for nurturing our inner microbial cosmos and fostering overall well-being.

CHAPTER THREE

NOURISHING YOUR GUT

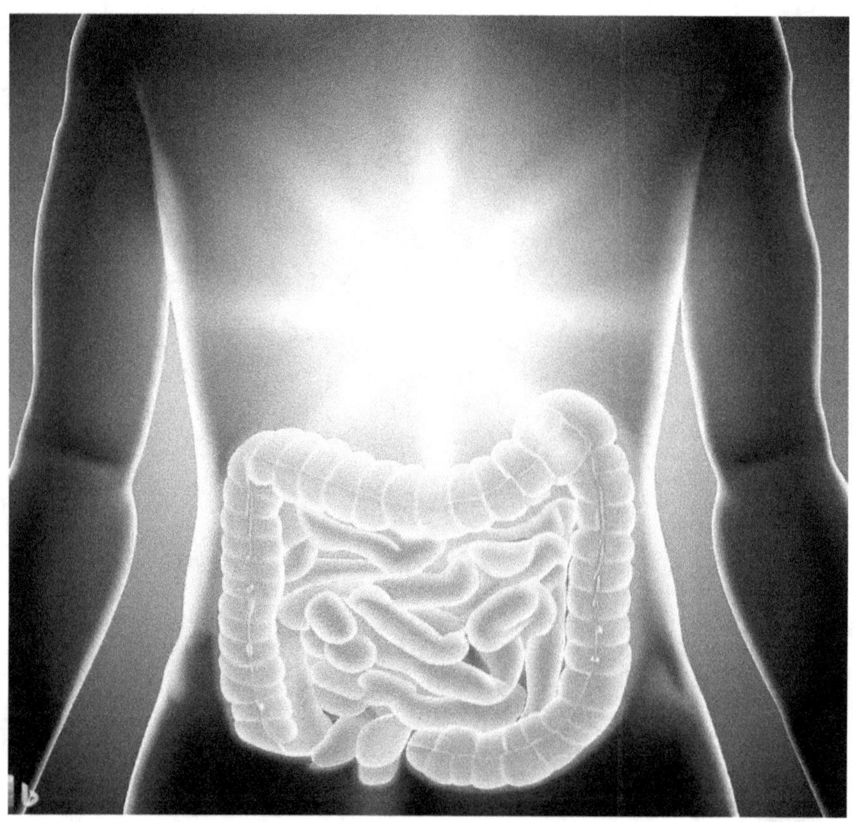

Gut nourishment is the practice of providing essential

nutrients and fostering a healthy environment within the

gastrointestinal tract to support overall well-being. It

recognizes the critical role that the gut plays in our health, serving as a hub for digestion, absorption of nutrients, and immune system regulation.

A well-nourished gut thrives on a balanced diet rich in fiber, prebiotics, and probiotics. Fiber, found in fruits, vegetables, and whole grains, supports regular bowel movements and feeds beneficial gut bacteria. Prebiotics, such as inulin and oligosaccharides, serve as food for these good bacteria, promoting their growth and activity. Probiotics, on the other hand, are live microorganisms that provide health benefits when consumed in adequate amounts. They help maintain a diverse and harmonious gut microbiome.

Moreover, gut nourishment extends beyond diet. Adequate hydration, stress management, and sufficient sleep are also integral to gut health. Chronic stress, poor sleep, and dehydration can disrupt the gut's delicate balance and contribute to gastrointestinal issues.

THE CLEAN GUT DIET: FOODS TO EMBRACE AND AVOID

The "Clean Gut" diet is a dietary approach designed to promote gut health by focusing on foods that support a balanced and flourishing gut microbiome while avoiding those that can disrupt it. Here's a guide to the foods you should embrace and avoid when following a Clean Gut Diet:

FOODS TO EMBRACE

Fiber-Rich Vegetables: Incorporate a variety of non-starchy vegetables like leafy greens, broccoli, cauliflower, and carrots. These provide essential nutrients and promote the growth of beneficial gut bacteria.

Fruits: Opt for low-sugar fruits such as berries, apples, and pears. They contain fiber, antioxidants, and polyphenols that support gut health.

Fermented Foods: Foods like yogurt, kefir, sauerkraut, kimchi, and kombucha are rich in probiotics, which introduce beneficial bacteria into the gut.

Prebiotic Foods: Prebiotics are non-digestible fibers that feed beneficial gut bacteria. Include foods like garlic, onions, leeks, and asparagus in your diet.

Lean Proteins: Choose lean sources of protein such as poultry, fish, tofu, and legumes. These provide amino acids without excessive fat.

Healthy Fats: Incorporate sources of healthy fats like avocados, olive oil, and nuts. These fats support gut health and reduce inflammation.

Bone Broth: Bone broth is rich in collagen and amino acids, which can help repair the gut lining.

Herbs and Spices: Turmeric, ginger, and oregano have anti-inflammatory properties and can be beneficial for gut health.

Probiotic Supplements: In some cases, probiotic supplements may be recommended by a healthcare provider to help restore a healthy gut microbiome.

FOODS TO AVOID

Processed Foods: Highly processed foods often contain additives, preservatives, and artificial sweeteners that can negatively impact gut health.

Added Sugars: Excessive sugar intake can promote the growth of harmful bacteria in the gut. Avoid sugary beverages, candies, and desserts.

Artificial Sweeteners: Some artificial sweeteners, like aspartame and saccharin, have been associated with gut dysbiosis and should be limited.

Refined Carbohydrates: White bread, pasta, and other refined carbohydrates can lead to spikes in blood sugar and negatively affect gut bacteria.

Saturated and Trans-Fats: High intake of saturated and trans-fats from fried foods and certain processed snacks can promote inflammation and disrupt gut health.

Dairy Products (for some): Some individuals are lactose intolerant or sensitive to dairy. If dairy causes digestive discomfort, it may be best to avoid it.

Alcohol: Excessive alcohol consumption can harm the gut lining and disrupt the gut microbiome. Moderate or eliminate alcohol consumption for optimal gut health.

Caffeine and Spicy Foods (for some): In some individuals, caffeine and very spicy foods can irritate the gastrointestinal tract. If you experience discomfort, consider reducing your intake.

Antibiotics (when not medically necessary): Overuse or unnecessary use of antibiotics can disrupt the gut microbiome. Only take antibiotics when prescribed by a healthcare professional.

Remember that individual responses to foods can vary, and what works best for one person may not be the same for another. It's often a good idea to consult with a healthcare provider or registered dietitian when making significant dietary changes, especially if you have specific digestive issues or health concerns.

MEAL PLANNING FOR GUT HEALTH

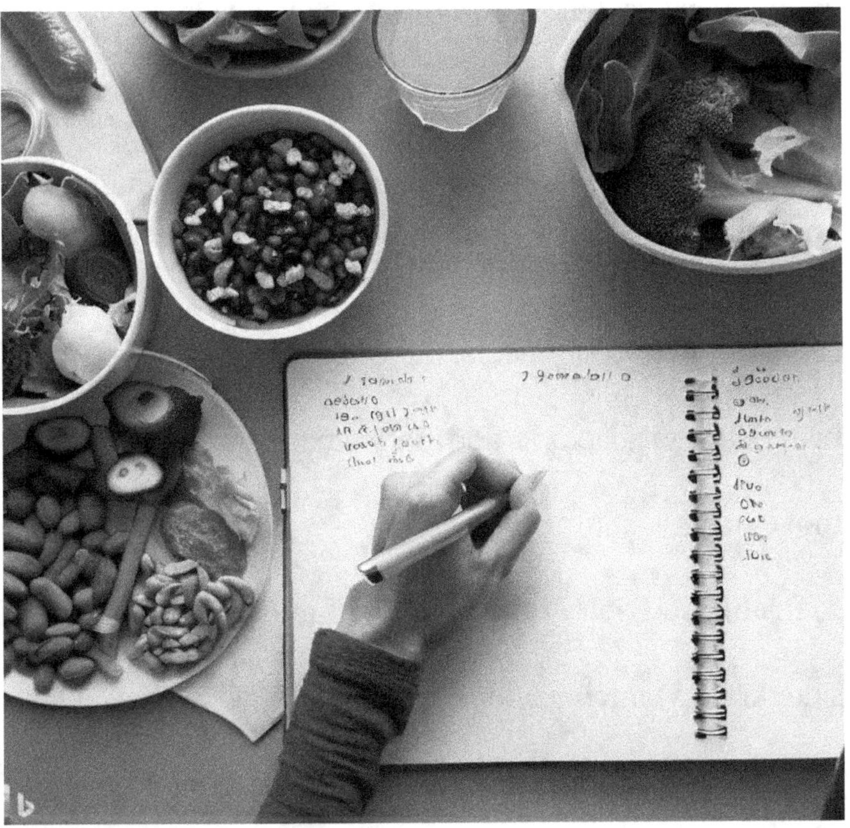

Meal planning for gut health involves making dietary choices that promote the well-being of your gastrointestinal tract. A healthy gut is linked to improved digestion, better nutrient absorption, a strong immune system, and even better mental health. Here's a comprehensive guide on how to plan meals for optimal gut health:

1. Prioritize Fiber: Incorporate a variety of high-fiber foods such as fruits, vegetables, whole grains, legumes, and nuts into your meals. Fiber supports the growth of beneficial gut bacteria and helps maintain regular bowel movements.

2. Probiotic-Rich Foods: Include foods like yogurt, kefir, sauerkraut, kimchi, and kombucha in your diet. These foods contain live beneficial bacteria (probiotics) that can enhance the microbial balance in your gut.

3. Prebiotics: Consume prebiotic-rich foods like garlic, onions, leeks, asparagus, and bananas. Prebiotics are non-digestible fibers that nourish the beneficial bacteria in your gut.

4. Lean Proteins: Opt for lean sources of protein like poultry, fish, tofu, and legumes. Excessive red meat consumption can negatively impact gut health.

5. Whole Grains: Choose whole grains like brown rice, quinoa, whole wheat, and oats over refined grains. Whole grains are rich in fiber and provide essential nutrients.

6. Healthy Fats: Incorporate sources of healthy fats, such as avocados, nuts, seeds, and olive oil. These fats support overall health, including gut health.

7. Limit Added Sugars: Reduce your intake of foods and beverages high in added sugars, as excessive sugar consumption can disrupt the balance of gut bacteria.

8. Fermented Foods: Integrate fermented foods into your diet regularly. Fermentation not only preserves food but also enhances its probiotic content. Examples include miso, tempeh, and pickles.

9. Stay Hydrated: Adequate hydration is crucial for digestion. Aim to drink plenty of water throughout the day.

10. Be Mindful of Food Sensitivities: Pay attention to how your body reacts to certain foods. If you suspect food sensitivities or allergies, consider an elimination diet to identify and avoid trigger foods.

11. Avoid Overuse of Antibiotics: Use antibiotics only when prescribed by a healthcare professional. Overuse can disrupt the balance of gut bacteria.

12. Practice Mindful Eating: Eating slowly and mindfully can aid digestion. Chew your food thoroughly and savor the flavors.

13. Manage Stress: Chronic stress can negatively affect gut health. Incorporate stress-reduction techniques like meditation, yoga, or deep breathing into your routine.

14. Plan Balanced Meals: Create meals that include a balance of carbohydrates, proteins, and fats. This balance can help maintain stable blood sugar levels and support overall health.

15. Variety is Key: Aim for a diverse diet. Different foods provide different nutrients and promote the growth of various beneficial gut bacteria.

SAMPLE MEAL PLAN

Breakfast:

Greek yogurt with berries and a sprinkle of chia seeds.

Whole-grain toast with avocado.

Lunch:

Grilled chicken salad with mixed greens, tomatoes, cucumbers, and a vinaigrette dressing.

A side of sautéed asparagus.

Snack:

A small handful of mixed nuts.

Dinner:

Baked salmon with a side of quinoa.

Steamed broccoli with garlic.

Dessert (occasional):

A small serving of dark chocolate.

Remember that individual dietary needs can vary. It's a good idea to consult with a healthcare provider or registered dietitian for personalized meal planning, especially if you have specific gut-related conditions or dietary restrictions. Regularly assessing how your body responds to different foods can also help you tailor your meal plan for optimal gut health.

CHAPTER FOUR

DIGESTIVE RESET:CLEANSE AND DETOX

GENTLE CLEANSING METHODS

Gentle cleansing methods can help support gut health without resorting to harsh or extreme measures. Here's a guide to some of the most effective and gentle approaches:

1. Dietary Fiber:

Increasing dietary fiber is one of the gentlest and most effective ways to support gut health. Fiber-rich foods, such as whole grains, fruits, vegetables, and legumes, promote regular bowel movements and provide nourishment for beneficial gut bacteria. The recommended daily intake of fiber is around 25-30 grams for adults, but individual needs may vary.

2. Hydration:

Adequate hydration is essential for a healthy gut. Water helps in the digestion and absorption of nutrients and keeps the mucosal lining of the intestines moist. Drinking enough water also prevents constipation, which can negatively impact gut health.

3. Probiotics and Prebiotics:

Probiotics are live beneficial bacteria, and prebiotics are compounds that nourish these bacteria. Including probiotic-rich foods like yogurt, kefir, sauerkraut, and kimchi in your diet can help maintain a balanced gut microbiome. Prebiotic foods like garlic, onions, leeks, and asparagus provide the necessary fuel for these friendly bacteria.

4. Slow and Mindful Eating:

Eating slowly and mindfully can aid digestion. Chewing your food thoroughly and savoring each bite allows for better breakdown of food in the stomach, making it easier for the gut to absorb nutrients. It can also reduce the risk of overeating, which can strain the digestive system.

5. Herbal Teas:

Certain herbal teas, such as ginger, peppermint, and chamomile, have soothing properties that can calm digestive discomfort. Ginger, in particular, is known for its anti-inflammatory and anti-nausea effects.

6. Gentle Exercise:

Regular, moderate exercise can promote gut health by enhancing digestion and reducing the risk of constipation. Activities like walking, yoga, and swimming are excellent choices.

7. Stress Management:

Chronic stress can negatively affect gut health by disrupting the balance of the gut microbiome. Practices like meditation, deep breathing exercises, and mindfulness can help reduce stress and support a healthy gut.

8. Limiting Processed Foods:

Highly processed foods often contain additives, preservatives, and artificial sweeteners that can disrupt the gut microbiome. Reducing your intake of processed foods and opting for whole, natural foods can be beneficial.

9. Elimination Diets with Professional Guidance:

In some cases, individuals with specific gut issues may benefit from elimination diets, such as FODMAP or gluten-free diets. However, it's essential to do these under the guidance of a healthcare professional or registered dietitian to ensure you're getting all the necessary nutrients.

10. Detoxification with Caution:

While various detox diets and cleanses are promoted for gut health, they should be approached with caution. Many of these plans lack scientific evidence and can be harsh on the body. It's advisable to consult a healthcare professional before attempting any detox regimen.

Remember, everyone's gut is unique, and what works for one person may not work the same way for another. It's essential to listen to your body, pay attention to how different foods and practices affect you, and consult a healthcare provider or registered dietitian if you have specific concerns or conditions related to gut health. Gentle, sustainable changes to your lifestyle and diet are often the most effective ways to support a healthy gut over the long term.

REVITALIZING GUT-FRIENDLY DETOX RECIPES

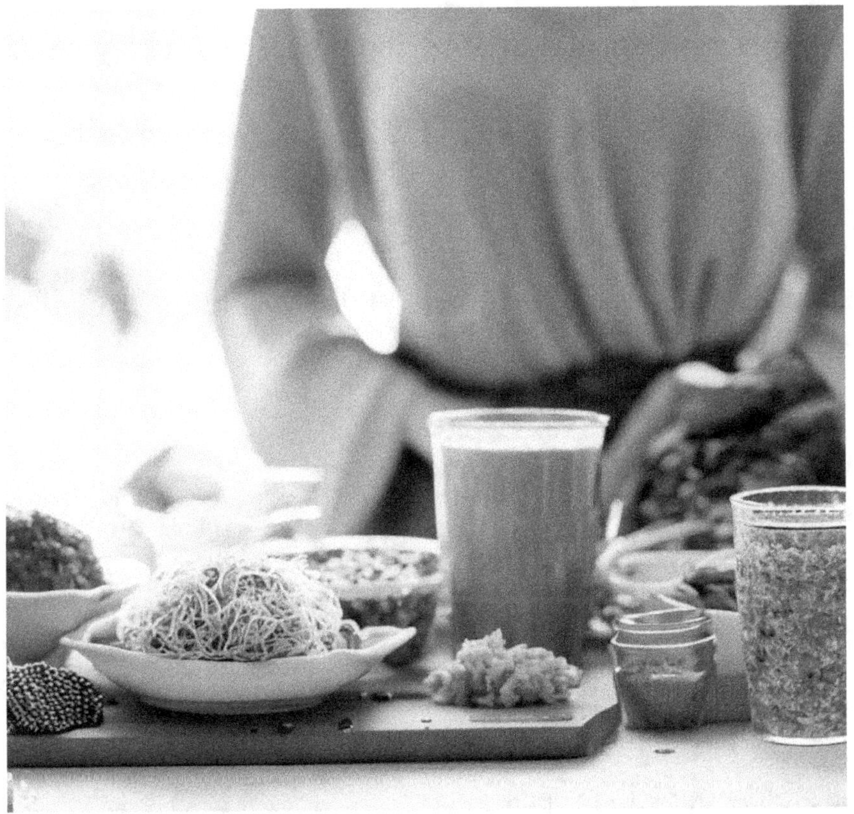

Detoxifying the body is a concept as old as time, rooted in the belief that cleansing from within can rejuvenate our health and vitality. While the science behind traditional detox diets is often debated, one aspect consistently agreed upon is that a diet rich in gut-friendly, nutrient-dense foods can support overall well-being. Here, we present a collection of revitalizing, gut-friendly detox recipes to help you kickstart a journey towards better health.

1. Green Smoothie Bowl: The Ultimate Morning Reviver

Ingredients:

1 cup spinach or kale leaves

1/2 cucumber, peeled and sliced

1/2 banana

1/2 cup unsweetened almond milk

1 tablespoon chia seeds

1 tablespoon honey or maple syrup (optional)

Fresh berries and sliced almonds for topping

Instructions:

Blend the spinach or kale, cucumber, banana, almond milk, chia seeds, and honey until smooth. Pour into a bowl and top with fresh berries and sliced almonds. This green smoothie bowl is packed with fiber, vitamins, and minerals to kickstart your day and support gut health.

2. Quinoa and Roasted Veggie Salad: Gut-Friendly Fiber Feast

Ingredients:

1 cup cooked quinoa

1 cup mixed roasted vegetables (e.g., bell peppers, zucchini, carrots)

1/4 cup chickpeas

2 tablespoons extra-virgin olive oil

1 tablespoon lemon juice

1 clove garlic, minced

Salt and pepper to taste

Fresh herbs (e.g., parsley, cilantro) for garnish

Instructions:

In a bowl, combine the cooked quinoa, roasted vegetables, and chickpeas. In a separate small bowl, whisk together the olive oil, lemon juice, minced garlic, salt, and pepper. Pour the dressing over the quinoa and veggie mixture. Garnish with fresh herbs. This fiber-rich salad promotes a healthy gut microbiome.

3. Turmeric and Ginger Detox Tea: Soothing Elixir

Ingredients:

1 cup hot water

1-inch piece of fresh ginger, sliced

1 teaspoon ground turmeric

1 teaspoon honey (optional)

Instructions:

Steep the fresh ginger and ground turmeric in hot water for 5-10 minutes. Strain, add honey if desired, and sip slowly. Both turmeric and ginger have anti-inflammatory properties and can soothe the digestive system.

4. Baked Salmon with Lemon and Dill: Omega-3 Powerhouse

Ingredients:

2 salmon fillets

1 lemon, thinly sliced

2 tablespoons fresh dill, chopped

2 cloves garlic, minced

Salt and pepper to taste

Olive oil for drizzling

Instructions:

Preheat your oven to 375°F (190°C). Place the salmon fillets on a baking sheet lined with parchment paper. Season with salt, pepper, and minced garlic. Top with lemon slices and chopped dill. Drizzle with olive oil. Bake for 15-20 minutes or until the salmon flakes easily with a fork. Salmon is rich in omega-3 fatty acids, which can benefit gut health and reduce inflammation.

5. Coconut Yogurt Parfait: Probiotic Delight

Ingredients:

1 cup coconut yogurt (or any probiotic-rich yogurt)

1/2 cup mixed berries (e.g., blueberries, strawberries)

1 tablespoon honey

2 tablespoons granola

Instructions:

Layer the coconut yogurt, mixed berries, honey, and granola in a glass or bowl. This parfait is a delicious way to introduce probiotics into your diet, promoting a healthy gut microbiome.

Remember, detoxing doesn't mean starving yourself. These gut-friendly recipes are designed to support your body's natural detoxification processes while providing essential nutrients and promoting a healthy gut. Incorporate these dishes into your diet to kickstart your journey toward improved well-being from the inside out.

CHAPTER FIVE

GUT-HEALING SUPPLEMENTS AND HERBS

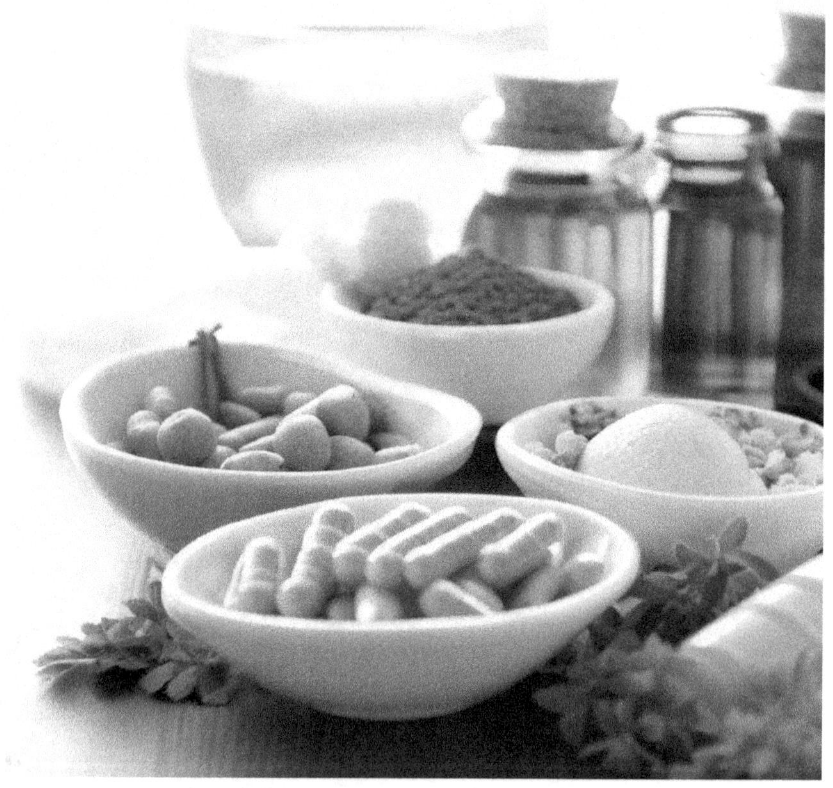

Gut-healing supplements and herbs have gained significant attention in recent years as people become more aware of the crucial role gut health plays in overall well-being. These supplements and herbs are often used to support and promote a healthy gut microbiome, alleviate gastrointestinal discomfort, and address conditions like irritable bowel syndrome (IBS) or leaky gut syndrome. However, it's important to approach them with knowledge and caution.

NATURAL REMEDIES FOR GUT RESTORATION

When the balance of this microbial community is disrupted, it can lead to various health issues. Fortunately, nature provides an array of natural remedies that can help restore and maintain gut health.

1. Dietary Fiber: The Gut's Best Friend

A diet rich in dietary fiber is essential for gut health. Fiber acts as a prebiotic, providing nourishment for beneficial gut bacteria. Foods like whole grains, legumes, fruits, and vegetables are excellent sources of dietary fiber. Incorporating these into your diet can promote a healthier gut microbiome.

2. Probiotic Foods: Replenishing the Good Bacteria

Probiotic foods are packed with beneficial live bacteria that can help restore the gut's microbial balance. Examples include yogurt, kefir, sauerkraut, kimchi, and kombucha. Regular consumption of these foods can introduce friendly bacteria into your gut.

3. Prebiotic Foods: Feeding the Good Bacteria

Prebiotics are non-digestible fibers found in certain foods that nourish and stimulate the growth of beneficial gut bacteria. Foods like garlic, onions, leeks, asparagus, and bananas contain prebiotics and can support a healthy gut microbiome.

4. Bone Broth: Gut Soothing Elixir

Bone broth is rich in collagen, amino acids, and minerals that can help heal and soothe the gut lining. It can be particularly beneficial for individuals with conditions like leaky gut syndrome. Homemade bone broth from grass-fed or organic sources is preferred for maximum benefits.

5. Fermented Foods: A Gut's Delight

Fermented foods are not only delicious but also great for gut health. Fermentation introduces beneficial bacteria into these foods, making them potent probiotics. Besides yogurt and kimchi, consider miso, tempeh, and traditional pickles in your diet.

6. Ginger and Turmeric: Natural Anti-Inflammatories

Ginger and turmeric possess anti-inflammatory properties that can help reduce gut inflammation and discomfort.

Incorporate them into your cooking or prepare soothing teas to support gut healing.

7. Aloe Vera: Soothing Gut Irritation

Aloe vera is well-known for its soothing properties. Drinking aloe vera juice, especially in its pure form, can help calm gastrointestinal irritation and inflammation.

8. Slippery Elm: Gentle Gut Healer

Slippery elm is an herb known for its mucilage content, which can coat and soothe the gut lining. It's available in various forms, including teas and supplements, and can be helpful for individuals with digestive issues.

9. Apple Cider Vinegar: Digestive Aid

Apple cider vinegar, when consumed in moderation, can support digestion by increasing stomach acid production. This can be particularly helpful for individuals with low stomach acid levels.

10. Stress Reduction: Mind-Gut Connection

Stress can negatively affect gut health by disrupting the balance of gut bacteria and increasing inflammation. Practices like meditation, yoga, and mindfulness can help manage stress and indirectly support gut restoration.

11. Hydration: A Fundamental Aspect

Staying adequately hydrated is essential for overall health, including gut function. Water helps maintain the mucosal lining of the intestines and supports digestion.

12. Sleep: The Gut's Restorative Partner

Quality sleep is crucial for gut health. It allows the body to repair and regenerate, including the gut lining. Aim for 7-9 hours of uninterrupted sleep each night.

Remember that everyone's gut is unique, and what works for one person may not work the same way for another. If you have specific gut health concerns or conditions, it's advisable to consult with a healthcare professional or a registered dietitian who can provide personalized guidance and recommendations tailored to your needs.

HOW TO USE SUPPLEMENTS SAFELY AND EFFECTIVELY

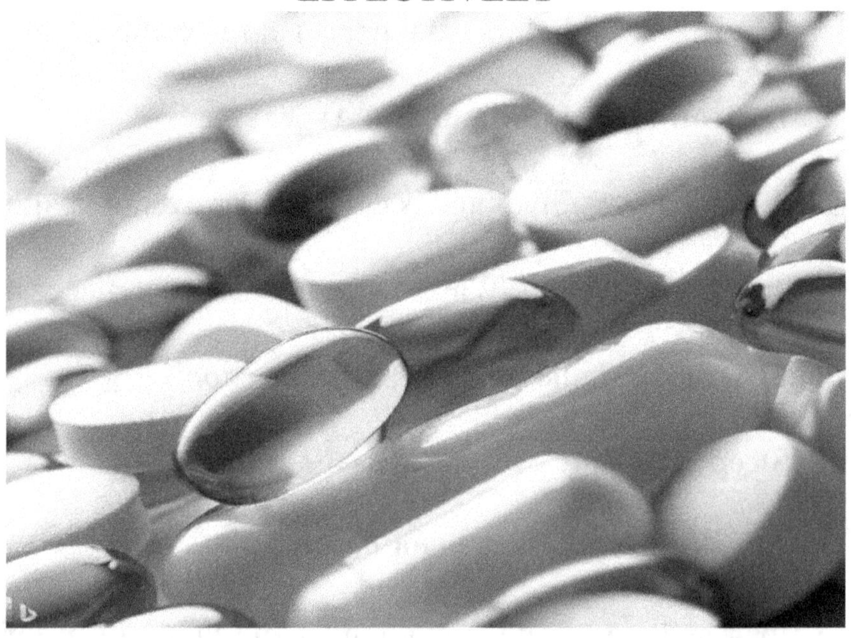

Using supplements safely and effectively is crucial for maintaining good health and achieving your fitness or wellness goals. Here are some key guidelines to follow:

1. Consult a Healthcare Professional:

Before starting any supplement regimen, consult with a healthcare provider, especially if you have underlying health conditions, are pregnant, nursing, or taking medications. They can help you determine if supplements are necessary and safe for you.

2. Choose Reputable Brands:

Purchase supplements from reputable companies that follow good manufacturing practices (GMP). Look for third-party testing and certifications to ensure quality and purity.

3. Understand Your Needs:

Identify your specific nutritional needs through a balanced diet and, if necessary, blood tests. Avoid taking supplements if you are already meeting your nutritional requirements through food.

4. Start with a Multivitamin:

If you're unsure where to begin, a basic multivitamin can provide a foundation of essential vitamins and minerals. However, remember that supplements should not be a substitute for a balanced diet.

5. Follow Recommended Dosages:

Always follow the recommended dosage on the supplement label. More is not necessarily better, and excessive intake can lead to adverse effects.

6. Be Cautious with Mega-Doses:

Avoid mega-doses of vitamins and minerals unless prescribed by a healthcare professional. High doses can be harmful and may interact with medications.

7. Pay Attention to Timing:

Some supplements are best taken with food, while others are better on an empty stomach. Read the instructions and follow them.

8. Take Fat-Soluble Vitamins with Fat:

Vitamins A, D, E, and K are fat-soluble, meaning they are absorbed better when taken with dietary fat. Consider taking them with a meal that contains healthy fats.

9. Monitor for Side Effects:

Pay attention to how your body responds to supplements. If you experience adverse effects like digestive problems, nausea, or skin reactions, discontinue use and consult your healthcare provider.

10. Be Patient:

Supplements often take time to show effects. Don't expect immediate results, and give them time to work in conjunction with a healthy lifestyle.

11. Be Consistent:

Consistency is key. Take your supplements regularly as recommended for the best results.

12. Avoid Herbal Interactions:

Be cautious when taking herbal supplements, as they can interact with medications or have unexpected side effects. Consult your healthcare provider if you're unsure.

13. Rotate Supplements:

If you take multiple supplements, consider rotating them to prevent overloading on any specific nutrient.

14. Store Properly:

Store supplements in a cool, dry place away from direct sunlight, and keep them out of reach of children.

15. Re-evaluate Regularly:

Periodically reassess your supplement regimen with your healthcare provider to ensure that it still meets your needs and is safe.

Remember that supplements should complement a healthy diet, not replace it. Whole foods provide a wide range of nutrients and other beneficial compounds that supplements cannot replicate. Strive for a balanced diet and use supplements as a backup when necessary.

CHAPTER SIX

MIND-GUT CONNECTION

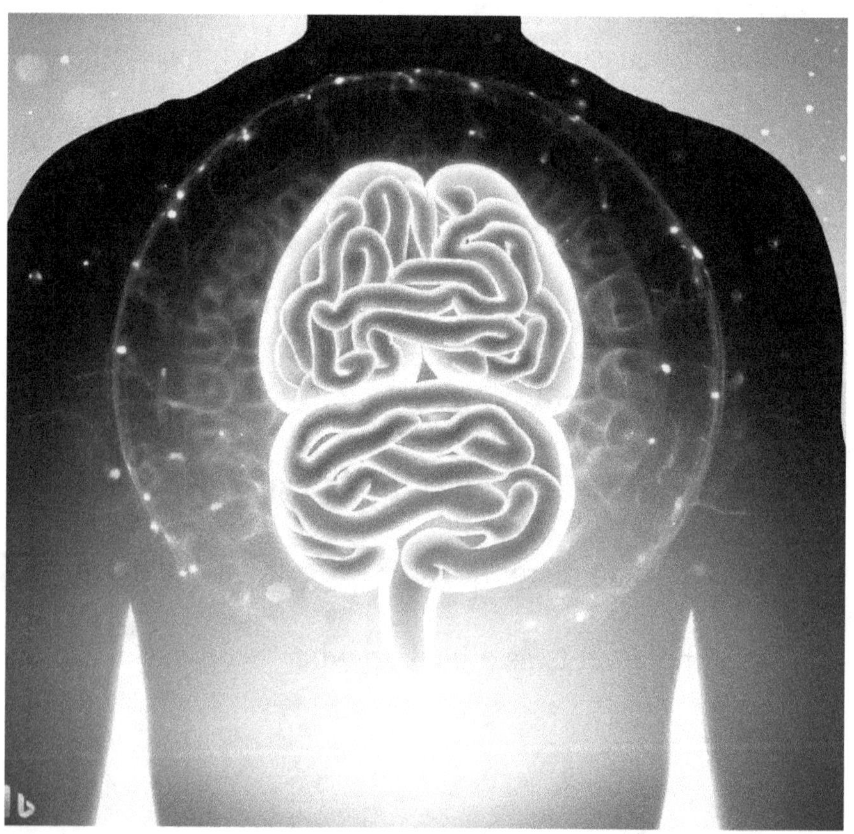

The "mind-gut connection" refers to the bidirectional communication between the brain (mind) and the gut (digestive system). This connection is a complex and dynamic relationship that involves various physiological and biochemical pathways, as well as the nervous system. Here are some key points about the mind-gut connection:

1. Enteric Nervous System (ENS): The gut has its own nervous system, known as the enteric nervous system (ENS). It consists of millions of neurons that regulate various gastrointestinal functions independently of the central nervous system (CNS). However, the ENS can also communicate with the brain through the vagus nerve.

2. Vagus Nerve: The vagus nerve is a major part of the autonomic nervous system that connects the brain to the gut. It plays a crucial role in transmitting information between the two. Signals travel up the vagus nerve from the gut to the brain and vice versa.

3. Neurotransmitters: The gut produces and houses several neurotransmitters, including serotonin, dopamine, and GABA, which are also present in the brain. These neurotransmitters play a role in mood regulation and may influence emotions and mental health.

4. Microbiome: The gut is home to trillions of microorganisms, collectively known as the gut microbiota. These microbes can produce molecules that affect the brain, potentially influencing mood, behavior, and even cognitive function. This bidirectional communication between the gut microbiome and the brain is an area of active research.

5. Psychological Impact: Stress, anxiety, and other psychological factors can have a significant impact on gut function. For example, stress can lead to digestive issues such as irritable bowel syndrome (IBS), and conversely, gastrointestinal problems can affect mood and mental health.

6. Clinical Implications: The mind-gut connection has led to growing interest in the field of psychogastroenterology. Researchers and healthcare providers are exploring how psychological interventions, such as cognitive-behavioral therapy and mindfulness, can help manage digestive disorders. Additionally, dietary changes and probiotics are being studied for their potential to improve mental health.

7. Holistic Health: Recognizing the mind-gut connection highlights the importance of a holistic approach to health. It suggests that physical well-being and mental well-being are interconnected and that addressing one aspect can positively or negatively impact the other.

In summary, the mind-gut connection underscores the intricate relationship between the brain and the digestive system, emphasizing the need to consider both physical and psychological factors when addressing issues related to gut health and mental health.

STRESS AND ITS IMPACT ON GUT HEALTH

Stress and gut health are closely interconnected, and chronic stress can have a significant impact on the gastrointestinal (GI) system. This connection is often referred to as the "gut-brain axis," which represents the bidirectional communication between the brain and the gut. Here's how stress affects gut health:

Altered Gut Motility: Stress can lead to changes in gut motility, causing either diarrhea or constipation. The gut has its own nervous system (the enteric nervous system), which can be influenced by stress hormones, such as cortisol, leading to these disturbances.

Changes in Gut Microbiota: Stress can alter the composition and diversity of the gut microbiota. It can lead to a decrease in beneficial bacteria and an increase in harmful bacteria, which may contribute to digestive issues and inflammation in the gut.

Increased Permeability: Chronic stress can lead to increased intestinal permeability, often referred to as "leaky gut." This allows substances that are normally confined to the digestive tract to enter the bloodstream, potentially triggering immune responses and inflammation.

Inflammation: Stress can promote inflammation in the gut. This chronic low-level inflammation can contribute to conditions such as irritable bowel syndrome (IBS) and inflammatory bowel disease (IBD).

Immune Function: Stress can weaken the immune system, making the gut more susceptible to infections and inflammatory conditions.

Appetite and Food Choices: Stress can also influence eating habits. Some people may overeat or consume unhealthy foods as a way to cope with stress, which can negatively affect gut health.

Vicious Cycle: The relationship between stress and gut health can form a vicious cycle. A stressed mind can lead to gut issues, which in turn can exacerbate stress, creating a feedback loop.

To promote better gut health in the face of stress, consider these strategies:

Stress Management: Practice stress-reduction techniques such as mindfulness, meditation, yoga, or deep breathing exercises to help manage stress.

Diet: Consume a balanced diet rich in fiber, fruits, vegetables, and probiotic-rich foods like yogurt and kefir. These can support a healthy gut microbiota.

Regular Exercise: Engage in regular physical activity, which can help reduce stress and promote healthy gut function.

Adequate Sleep: Prioritize getting enough quality sleep, as lack of sleep can exacerbate both stress and gut issues.

Limit Alcohol and Caffeine: Excessive alcohol and caffeine consumption can aggravate gut problems, especially in the presence of stress.

Seek Professional Help: If you're experiencing chronic stress and digestive issues, it's essential to consult a healthcare provider. They can provide guidance on managing stress and may recommend treatments or therapies to address gut health problems.

In conclusion, stress can have a profound impact on gut health through various mechanisms. Managing stress and adopting a gut-friendly lifestyle can help mitigate these effects and promote overall well-being.

TECHNIQUES FOR REDUCING STRESS AND PROMOTING GUT BALANCE

Reducing stress and promoting gut balance are both important for overall health and well-being. There is a strong connection between the gut and the brain, often referred to as the gut-brain axis, which means that managing stress can positively impact gut health, and a healthy gut can, in turn, help reduce stress. Here are some techniques to achieve both goals:

1. Mindfulness and Meditation:

Practicing mindfulness and meditation can help reduce stress by calming the mind and promoting relaxation. This, in turn, can have a positive impact on your gut health.

2. Deep Breathing Exercises:

Deep breathing techniques, such as diaphragmatic breathing or the 4-7-8 technique, can help lower stress levels and reduce inflammation in the gut.

3. Regular Exercise:

Engaging in regular physical activity is known to reduce stress hormones like cortisol. Exercise can also promote gut health by enhancing gut motility and diversity of gut microbes.

4. Adequate Sleep:

Prioritize getting enough quality sleep as poor sleep patterns can contribute to stress and disrupt gut balance. Aim for 7-9 hours of sleep per night.

5. Balanced Diet:

Consume a diet rich in fiber, fruits, vegetables, and fermented foods like yogurt, kefir, and sauerkraut. These foods promote a healthy gut microbiome, which is linked to reduced stress and improved mental health.

6. Probiotics and Prebiotics:

Consider incorporating probiotics (live beneficial bacteria) and prebiotics (fiber-rich foods that nourish these bacteria) into your diet to support gut health. Always consult a healthcare professional before starting any new supplements.

7. Hydration:

Staying well-hydrated is essential for overall health, including gut health. Water helps transport nutrients and supports the mucous lining of the gut.

8. Limit Alcohol and Caffeine:

Excessive alcohol and caffeine consumption can disrupt gut health and increase stress. Moderation is key.

9. Manage Stress:

Stress management techniques such as yoga, tai chi, journaling, or talking to a therapist can be beneficial for both mental well-being and gut health.

10. Avoid Overeating and Mindful Eating:

Overeating can strain the digestive system. Practice mindful eating by paying attention to your body's hunger and fullness cues.

11. Avoid Trigger Foods:

Identify and avoid foods that may trigger digestive discomfort or inflammation in your gut, as they can contribute to stress.

12. Seek Professional Help:

If you have persistent gut issues or chronic stress, consult with a healthcare provider or a registered dietitian. They can offer personalized guidance and recommendations.

Remember that the relationship between stress and gut health is complex and can vary from person to person. It's essential to adopt a holistic approach to health that includes physical, mental, and dietary strategies to promote overall well-being and gut balance.

CHAPTER SEVEN

EXERCISE AND GUT HEALTH

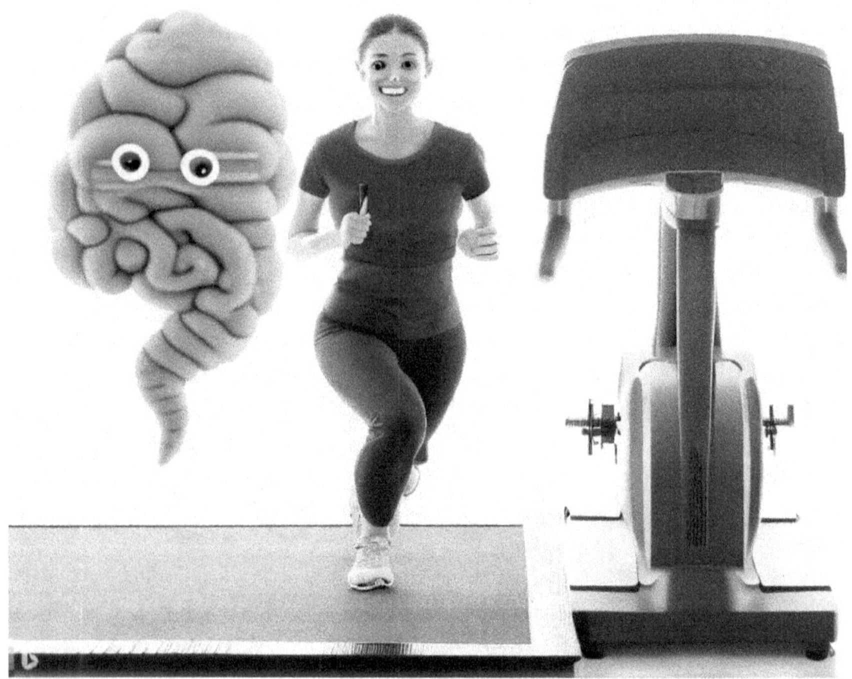

Exercise and gut health are closely linked, and the relationship between the two is a topic of growing interest in the field of health and wellness. Here's a brief discussion of their relationship:

Improved Gut Microbiota: Regular exercise can positively influence the composition and diversity of the gut microbiota. A diverse and balanced microbiome is associated with better overall health, including improved digestion and immune function.

Reduced Gut Inflammation: Exercise has anti-inflammatory effects on the body, which can extend to the gut. Chronic inflammation in the gut is linked to various digestive disorders, and exercise may help mitigate this inflammation.

Enhanced Bowel Regularity: Physical activity can stimulate bowel movements and alleviate constipation. It can help maintain healthy bowel function by promoting the rhythmic contractions of the intestines.

Weight Management: Exercise is crucial for weight management, and maintaining a healthy weight is essential for gut health. Obesity is linked to an increased risk of various gut-related issues, including gastroesophageal reflux disease (GERD) and irritable bowel syndrome (IBS).

Stress Reduction: Exercise is known to reduce stress, and stress can negatively impact gut health. High-stress levels can lead to changes in gut motility and gut microbiota composition.

Immune System Support: Regular physical activity can boost the immune system, which plays a significant role in maintaining a healthy gut. A strong immune system can help defend against infections and maintain gut homeostasis.

Butyrate Production: Exercise can increase the production of short-chain fatty acids like butyrate in the gut. Butyrate is beneficial for gut health as it helps nourish the cells lining the colon and may have protective effects against colorectal cancer.

Adaptation to Dietary Changes: Regular exercise can help the body adapt to changes in diet. This adaptability can be beneficial when transitioning to a diet that promotes gut health, such as one rich in fiber and fermented foods.

It's important to note that while exercise can have many positive effects on gut health, individual responses may vary. Additionally, excessive or very intense exercise may have negative consequences on gut health in some cases, so it's essential to strike a balance and consult with a healthcare professional if you have specific concerns about your gut health and exercise regimen.

PHYSICAL ACTIVITY FOR A HEALTHY GUT

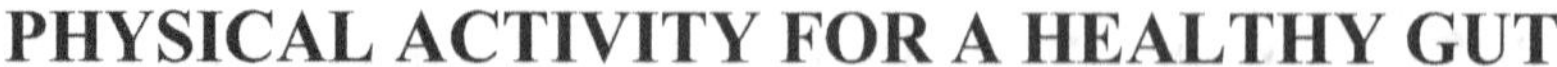

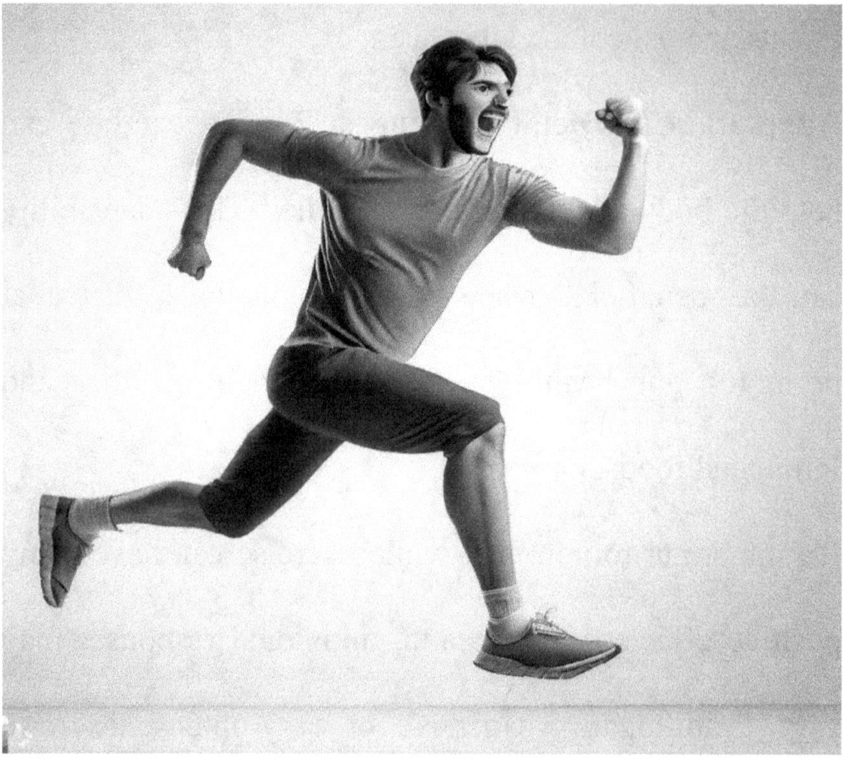

Physical activity plays a crucial role in maintaining overall health, including the health of your gut. A healthy gut is essential for proper digestion, nutrient absorption, and even immune function. Here's what you need to know about how physical activity can benefit your gut and the types of exercises that are effective for gut health:

1. Improved Gut Motility:

What: Physical activity helps to stimulate the muscles in your digestive tract, promoting regular bowel movements and preventing constipation.

Effective Activities: Aerobic exercises such as walking, jogging, cycling, and swimming can help improve gut motility.

2. Reduced Inflammation:

What: Chronic inflammation in the gut is associated with various digestive disorders. Regular exercise can help reduce overall inflammation in the body, including the gut.

Effective Activities: Both aerobic exercises and strength training can help reduce inflammation. Yoga and stretching exercises may also have anti-inflammatory effects.

3. Balanced Gut Microbiota:

What: A diverse and balanced gut microbiota is essential for digestive health. Exercise can positively influence the composition of your gut bacteria.

Effective Activities: While any form of exercise can potentially benefit gut microbiota, some studies suggest that high-intensity interval training (HIIT) and endurance exercise may be particularly effective.

4. Stress Reduction:

What: High stress levels can negatively impact gut health. Exercise is an excellent stress-reliever, which can indirectly benefit your gut.

Effective Activities: Activities like yoga, Pilates, and meditation, in addition to aerobic exercises, are excellent for stress reduction.

5. Weight Management:

What: Maintaining a healthy weight is crucial for gut health. Regular physical activity can help with weight management.

Effective Activities: A combination of aerobic exercises and strength training can be effective for weight management. Additionally, activities like hiking and dancing can be fun ways to stay active.

6. Enhanced Blood Flow:

What: Good blood circulation is vital for the health of all organs, including the gut. Exercise improves blood flow, which can benefit gut function.

Effective Activities: Any exercise that increases your heart rate and gets your blood pumping, such as brisk walking or jogging, can improve blood flow.

7. Hormone Regulation:

What: Exercise helps regulate hormones in the body, which can influence gut health. Hormonal imbalances can contribute to digestive issues.

Effective Activities: Regular, moderate-intensity exercise can help regulate hormones. Activities like cycling and swimming are good options.

8. Regularity and Consistency:

What: Consistency is key to reaping the gut health benefits of exercise. Aim for a regular workout routine.

Effective Activities: Choose exercises you enjoy to increase the likelihood of sticking with your routine.

Important Tips:

Stay hydrated before, during, and after exercise to support digestion.

Listen to your body. If you have a medical condition or experience digestive discomfort during exercise, consult a healthcare professional.

A balanced diet is also essential for gut health. Pair exercise with a diet rich in fiber, fruits, vegetables, and fermented foods for optimal results.

Remember that the key to gut health is balance. Over-exercising or pushing yourself too hard can have the opposite effect on your gut, so always aim for a balanced approach to physical activity that suits your individual fitness level and needs.

GUT-FRIENDLY WORKOUT ROUTINES

A gut-friendly workout routine focuses on exercises that can help improve digestion, reduce bloating, and strengthen the core muscles that support your digestive system. Here's a weekly timetable with recommended workout routines for a healthy gut:

Day 1: Yoga for Digestion

Morning: Start your week with a gentle yoga session. Yoga poses like Child's Pose, Cat-Cow, and Wind-Relieving Pose can help stimulate digestion and reduce bloating.

Day 2: Cardiovascular Exercise

Morning or Evening: Engage in 30-45 minutes of moderate-intensity cardio exercise such as brisk walking, cycling, or swimming. Cardio workouts help boost metabolism and keep your digestive system active.

Day 3: Core Strengthening

Morning: Focus on core-strengthening exercises. Include planks, Russian twists, and leg raises in your routine. A strong core supports your digestive organs.

Day 4: Pilates for Gut Health

Morning: Try a Pilates workout. Pilates exercises like the Hundred and the Pilates Scissor can help improve core strength and digestion.

Day 5: Rest or Gentle Activity

***Morning or Evening*:** Take a break or engage in a low-intensity activity like walking or gentle stretching. Rest is essential for overall gut health.

Day 6: HIIT for Digestive Health

Morning: High-Intensity Interval Training (HIIT) can boost metabolism and promote digestion. Include exercises like burpees, mountain climbers, and squat jumps.

Day 7: Stretch and Relax

Morning: End your week with a restorative yoga or stretching session. Poses like Downward Dog and Cobra can help alleviate digestive discomfort.

Additional Tips:

- Stay hydrated throughout the week. Proper hydration is crucial for a healthy gut.

- Maintain a balanced diet with plenty of fiber-rich foods like fruits, vegetables, and whole grains.

- Practice mindful eating. Chew your food thoroughly and eat slowly to aid digestion.

- Avoid heavy, large meals close to bedtime.

This weekly workout timetable combines different forms of exercise to support digestive health. Remember that consistency is key, and it's important to choose activities that you enjoy and that align with your fitness level. Additionally, always consult with a healthcare professional before starting a new exercise program, especially if you have any underlying health conditions.

CHAPTER EIGHT

SLEEP AND GUT HEALTH

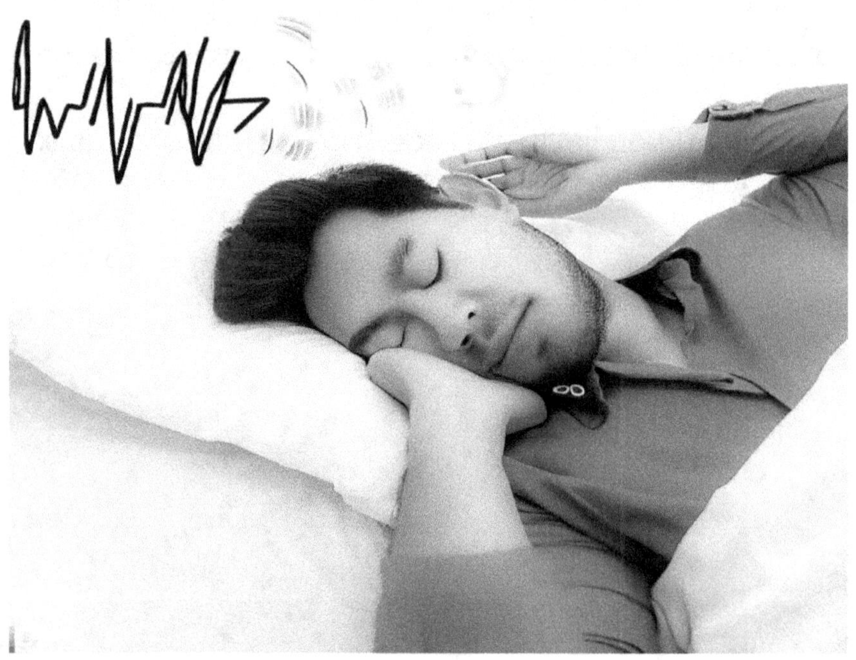

The connection between sleep and gut health is a fascinating and increasingly recognized aspect of human biology. Here's a brief background with some intriguing facts that might amaze you:

1. The Gut-Brain Axis:

Your gut and brain are in constant communication through a complex network of nerves, hormones, and chemicals. This bidirectional connection is known as the gut-brain axis.

This communication system influences not only digestion but also mood, stress, and even sleep.

2. Gut Microbiome and Sleep:

The gut is home to trillions of micro-organisms, collectively known as the gut microbiome. These microbes play a crucial role in digestion and overall health.

Emerging research suggests that the gut microbiome can also impact sleep patterns. The balance of "good" and "bad" bacteria in your gut may affect the quality and duration of your sleep.

3. Serotonin Production:

Serotonin, often called the "feel-good" neurotransmitter, is primarily produced in the gut. It helps regulate mood and sleep-wake cycles.

When your gut microbiome is out of balance, it can potentially lead to serotonin imbalances, which may contribute to sleep disturbances and mood disorders.

4. Circadian Rhythm Regulation:

Your circadian rhythm is your body's internal clock that regulates sleep and wake cycles. It's influenced by external cues like light and temperature.

Recent studies have shown that disruptions in the gut microbiome can disrupt the circadian rhythm, potentially leading to sleep problems.

5. Gut-Related Sleep Disorders:

Some sleep disorders are directly linked to gut health. For example, conditions like irritable bowel syndrome (IBS) are often accompanied by poor sleep quality. Conversely, chronic sleep deprivation can negatively impact the gut by altering its microbiome and increasing the risk of digestive disorders.

6. The Role of Diet:

What you eat can profoundly impact both your gut health and your sleep. Diets high in fiber, fruits, vegetables, and pro-biotics can promote a healthy gut and better sleep. Conversely, diets high in sugar and processed foods can disrupt the balance of gut bacteria and lead to sleep disturbances.

Intriguingly, this emerging field of research suggests that taking steps to improve your gut health, such as maintaining a balanced diet and managing stress, could have positive effects on your sleep quality and overall well-being. So, a good night's sleep might just start in your gut!

STRATEGIES FOR IMPROVING SLEEP QUALITY

Improving sleep quality is essential for overall health and well-being. Here are some pragmatic steps and strategies to help you get a better night's sleep:

1. Create a Consistent Sleep Schedule:

Go to bed and wake up at the same time every day, even on weekends. This helps regulate your body's internal clock.

2. Create a Relaxing Bedtime Routine:

Develop a calming pre-sleep routine to signal to your body that it's time to wind down. This could include activities like reading, gentle stretching, or taking a warm bath.

3. Optimize Your Sleep Environment:

Make your bedroom conducive to sleep. Keep it cool, dark, and quiet. Invest in a comfortable mattress and pillows.

Remove electronic devices, such as phones and tablets, from the bedroom, as the blue light emitted can interfere with your sleep.

4. Watch Your Diet:

Avoid heavy or large meals within a few hours of bedtime. These can cause discomfort and disrupt sleep.

Limit caffeine and alcohol intake, especially in the evening.

5. Get Regular Exercise:

Engage in regular physical activity, but try to finish exercising at least a few hours before bedtime. Exercise can help you fall asleep faster and enjoy deeper sleep.

6. Manage Stress:

Practice stress-reduction techniques such as meditation, deep breathing, or progressive muscle relaxation.

Consider keeping a journal to jot down worries and tasks for the next day to clear your mind before sleep.

7. Limit Screen Time Before Bed:

The blue light emitted by screens can interfere with the production of melatonin, a hormone that regulates sleep. Try to avoid screens at least an hour before bedtime.

8. Be Mindful of Naps:

While short power naps can be rejuvenating, long daytime naps can disrupt night-time sleep. If you nap, limit them to 20-30 minutes and earlier in the day.

9. Manage Your Bedroom Clock:

If you find yourself frequently checking the time during the night, consider turning your clock away from your line of sight. This can reduce anxiety about sleeplessness.

10. Seek Natural Light Exposure:

Exposure to natural light during the day helps regulate your circadian rhythm. Spend time outdoors during daylight hours.

11. Limit Fluid Intake Before Bed:

To reduce night-time awakenings to use the bathroom, avoid drinking large quantities of fluids close to bedtime.

12. Consider Professional Help:

If you've tried these strategies and continue to have sleep problems, consider consulting a sleep specialist or healthcare provider to rule out any underlying sleep disorders.

Remember, improving sleep quality often requires patience and persistence. It may take some time for your body to adjust to new habits and routines. Be consistent in your efforts, and over time, you should notice improvements in your sleep patterns and overall well-being.

CHAPTER NINE

BUILDING A GUT-HEALTHY LIFESTYLE

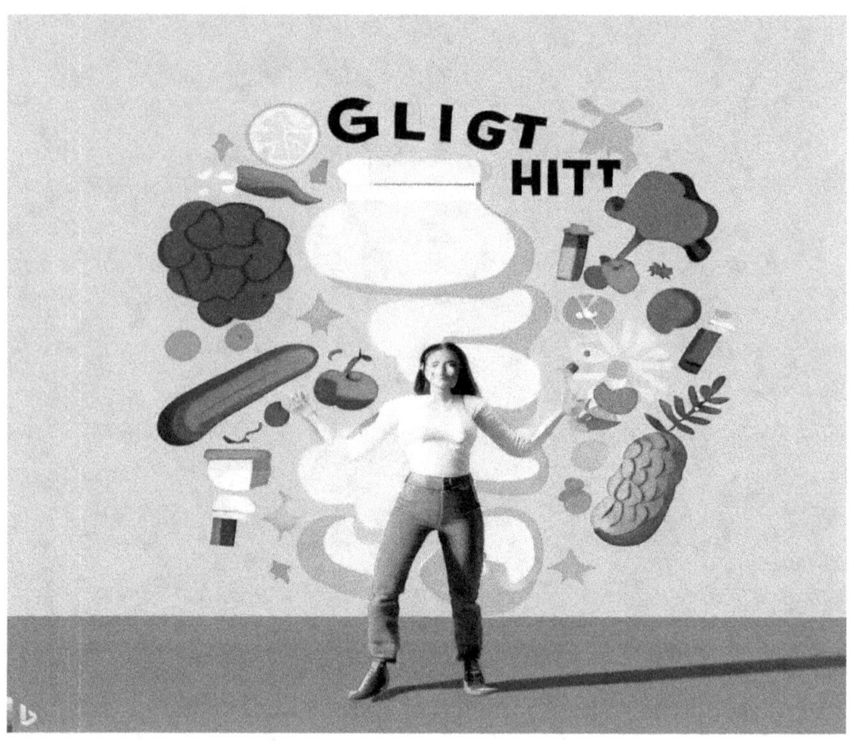

Your gut health is not just a matter of digestion; it's the cornerstone of your overall well-being. It influences your energy levels, mood, immune system, and even your sleep quality. Maintaining a clean and healthy gut is a journey that deserves your attention and dedication. Here's a call to action to inspire you on your gut health journey:

1. Embrace the Power of Your Plate:

Every meal is an opportunity to nourish your gut. Choose whole, unprocessed foods that are rich in fiber, vitamins, and minerals.

Incorporate probiotic-rich foods like yogurt, kefir, and sauerkraut to support a diverse gut microbiome.

2. Fiber is Your Friend:

Fiber is the foundation of a healthy gut. It supports regular bowel movements and provides essential nourishment for your gut bacteria.

Make it a goal to increase your fiber intake through fruits, vegetables, whole grains, and legumes.

3. Manage Stress Mindfully:

Chronic stress can wreak havoc on your gut health. Practice stress-reduction techniques like meditation, yoga, or deep breathing to keep your gut calm and balanced.

4. Prioritize Sleep:

Quality sleep is when your body does significant repair work, including maintaining your gut lining and microbiome.

Make sleep a priority in your life. Establish a consistent sleep schedule and create a sleep-friendly environment.

5. Move Your Body:

Exercise isn't just for the body; it's for your gut too. Regular physical activity supports digestion and reduces inflammation.

Find activities you enjoy to make exercise a sustainable part of your routine.

6. Listen to Your Gut:

Pay attention to how your gut feels after meals and in different situations. It can be a powerful indicator of your overall health.

If you experience persistent digestive issues, consult a healthcare professional for guidance.

7. Be Patient and Persistent:

Improving and maintaining gut health is a journey, not a destination. It takes time and consistency.

Celebrate small victories and stay committed to your long-term well-being.

8. Educate Yourself:

Knowledge is a potent tool in your gut health arsenal. Stay informed about the latest research and trends in gut health.

Understand that what works for one person may not work for another; your gut is unique.

9. Support and Accountability:

Consider sharing your gut health journey with friends or joining support groups. Having a support system can help you stay motivated.

Hold yourself accountable for your choices, and remember that your actions today shape your gut health tomorrow.

Your gut is a remarkable ecosystem, and caring for it is an act of self-love. By nurturing your gut health, you're investing in a healthier, happier, and more vibrant future. So, let this call to action be the catalyst for your sustained commitment to a clean and thriving gut, and ultimately, a more fulfilling life. Start today; your gut will thank you tomorrow.

....

Special note to the reader:

Dr. Chris Allan
Wishes you good health!